The Blood, Sweat, Tears, Tears, and Sweetness

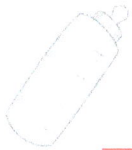

The Shit They Don't Tell You About Labor, Delivery, and The First 48 Hours Afterwards.

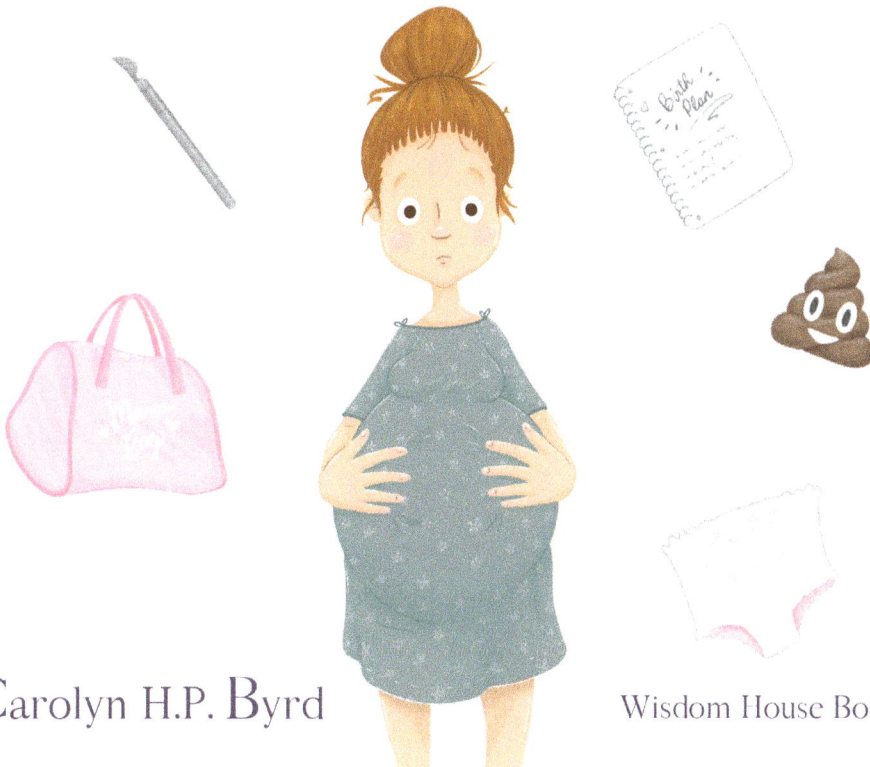

Carolyn H.P. Byrd

Wisdom House Books

The Blood, Sweat, Tears, Tears, and Sweetness

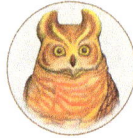

Published by Wisdom House Books, Inc.
Chapel Hill, North Carolina 27514 USA
www.wisdomhousebooks.com
Wisdom House Books is committed to excellence in the publishing industry.
Book design copyright © 2022 by Wisdom House Books, Inc.
All rights reserved.

Cover and Interior Illustration by Sarah Gramelspacher
Cover and Interior design by Ted Ruybal
Published in the United States of America
Hardback ISBN: 978-1-7363079-1-5
LCCN: 2022900143

1. HEA041000 | HEALTH & FITNESS / Pregnancy & Childbirth
2. FAM032000 | FAMILY & RELATIONSHIPS / Parenting / Motherhood
3. MED033000 | MEDICAL / Gynecology & Obstetrics

First Edition

25 24 23 22 21 20 / 10 9 8 7 6 5 4 3 2 1

Congratulations!

You did it! Yay!

You're in the homestretch and your baby is going to make its entrance into the world soon!

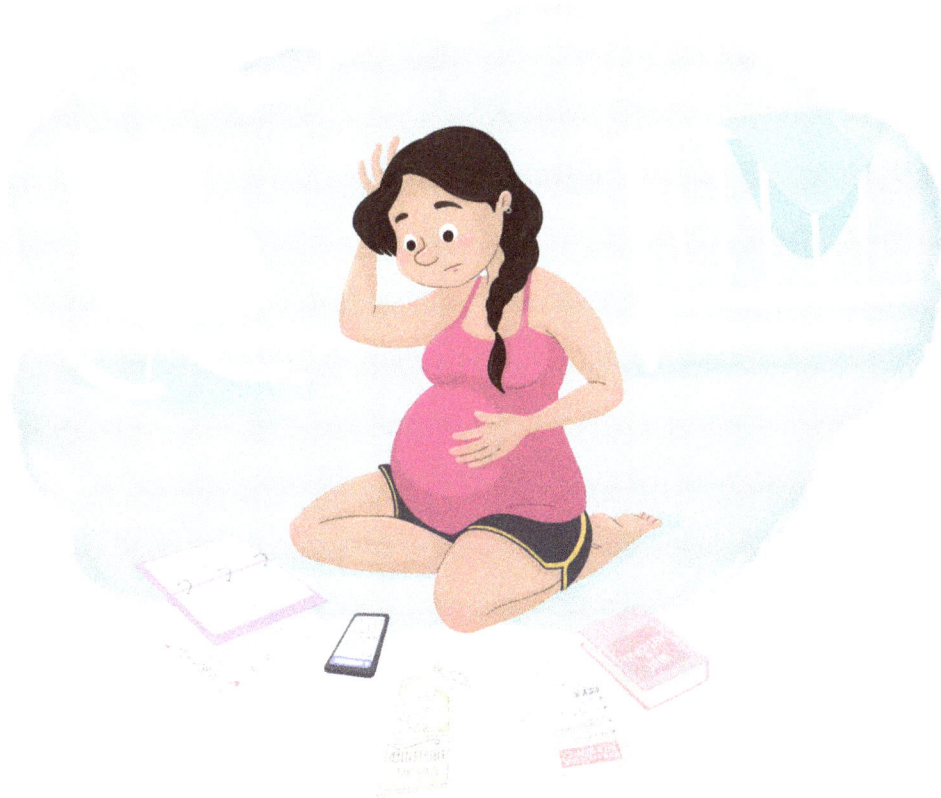

Being Ready

With the likes of backache, boob aches, swelling, health issues, and moving around like a barge you, mostly likely, will be ready to give your little one an eviction notice three to five weeks leading up to D-day.

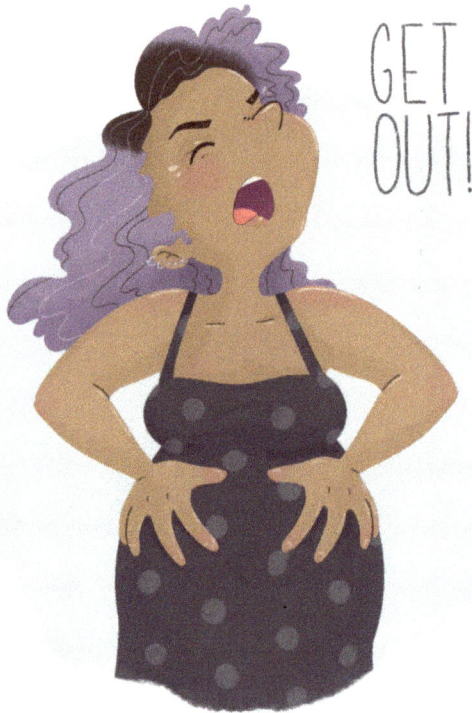

But not Quite Ready

Or you may relish the intimacy of being pregnant
and hope for some more time. Either is okay!

You're about to meet your little one, and that can spark
feelings on both sides.

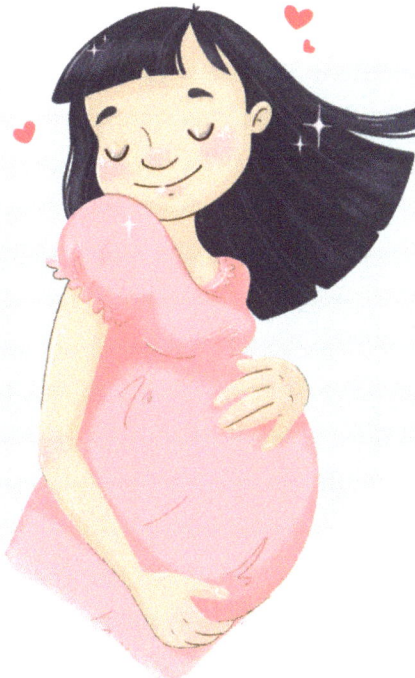

Braxton Hicks
and Prodromal Contractions

Your body will be getting ready for the big day, too, practicing labor with little, or big, contractions.

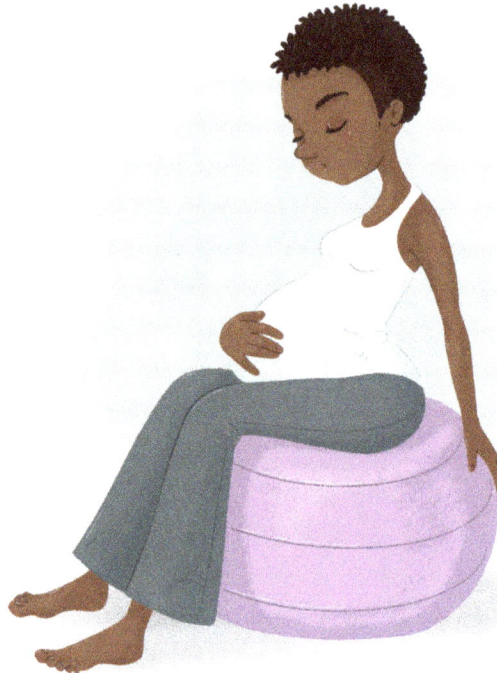

Fundal Massages

Massages down there can help prepare the tissue for delivery.

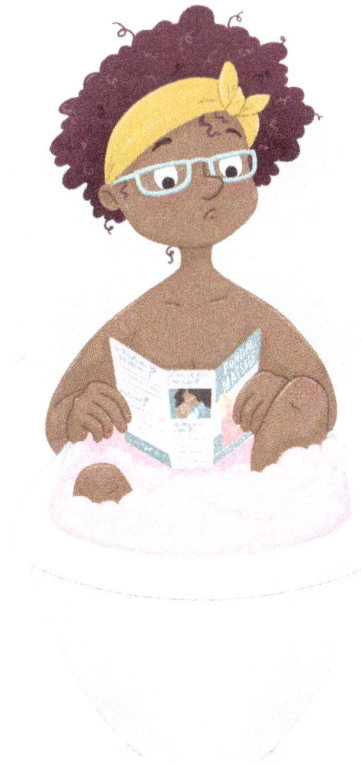

Don't Forget Dad, Partner, or Spouse

If you have a spouse or partner, include them in planning for the big day. This is for them too.

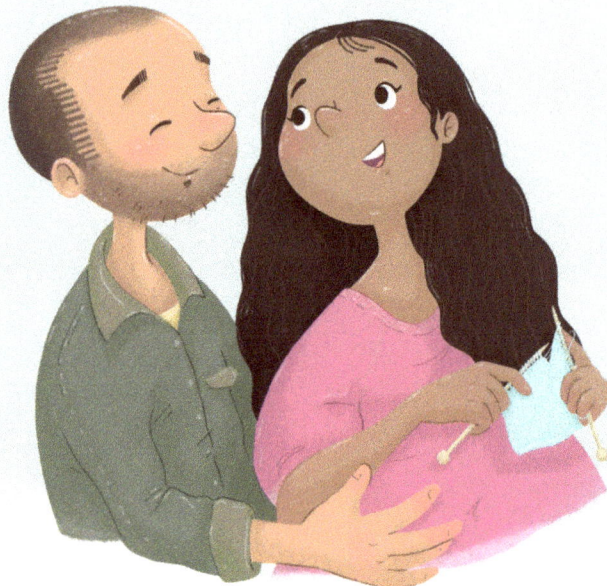

Birth Plans

Your labor and delivery experience may go exactly as planned
. . . or go to pot.

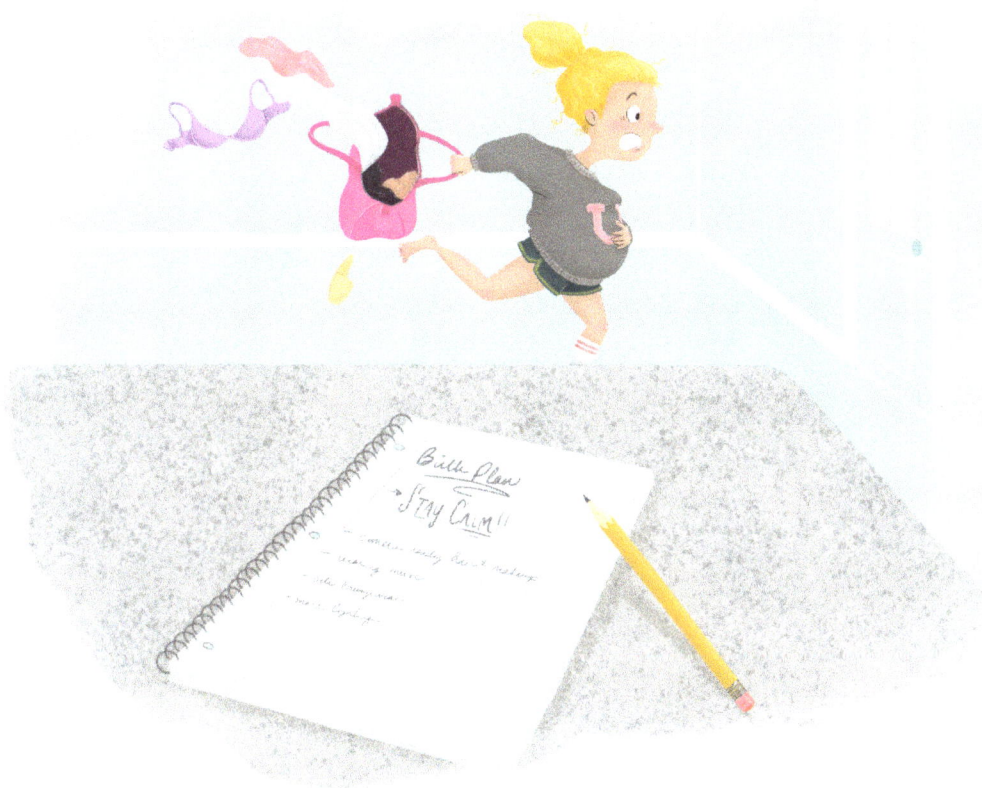

Doulas and Midwives

A doula or midwife can be very helpful.
Just be sure they have a good understanding of your wishes
and how to best support you.

As wonderful and knowledgeable as they can be,
it's your birth experience!

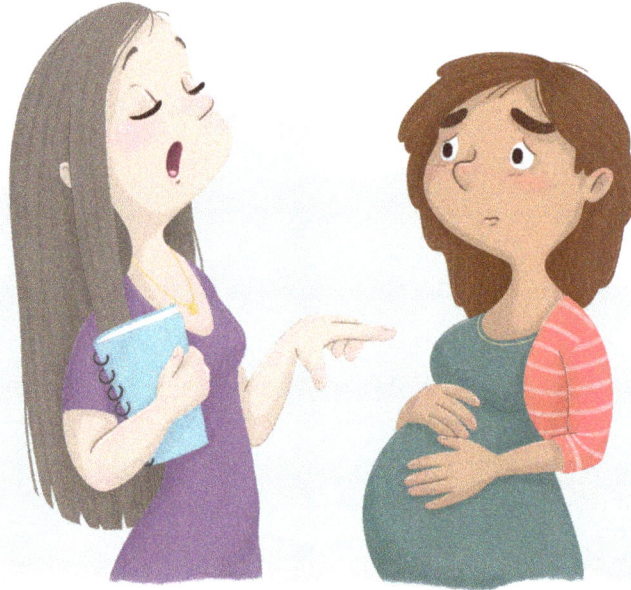

Pack for Comfort and Cuteness

It's your big day!

What is going to make you feel the most comfortable before, during, and after? Bring it!

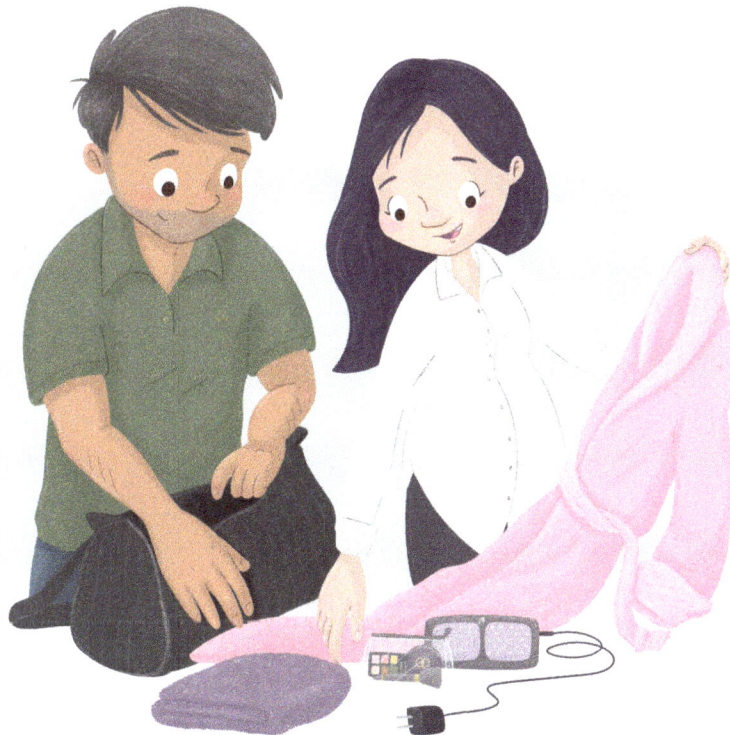

Due Date

. . . and when is that day happening?!

Well, your due date is a calculated guess,
plus or minus two weeks, at best.

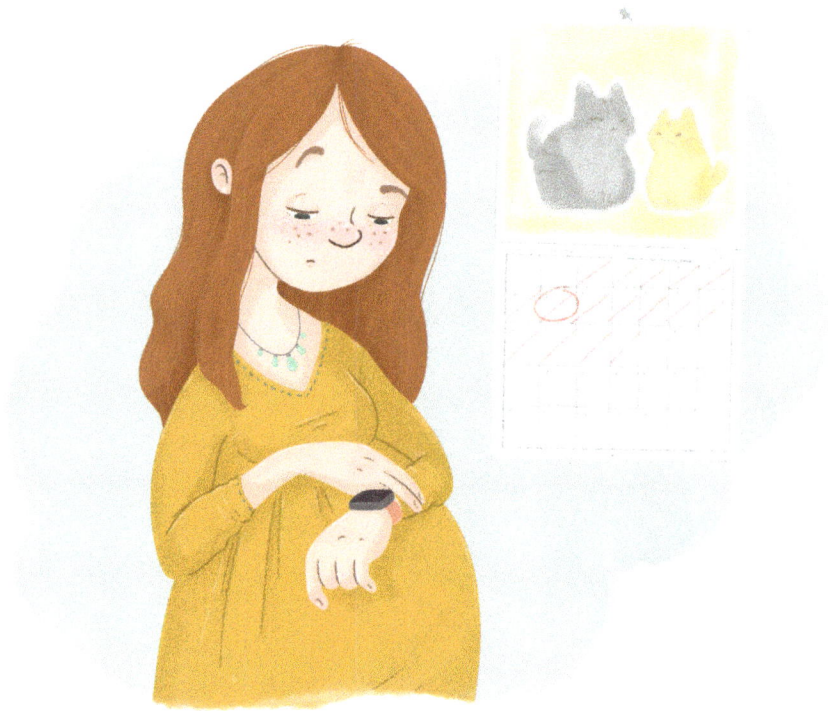

Tricks to Induce Labor

Walking, spicy foods, dates, and primrose oil are among some of the common labor inducing tricks.

Surprisingly, nipple stimulation may give an extra boost, too. It is said to release oxytocin which is a naturally occurring labor-inducing chemical.

However, sex is known to be one of the best ways to induce labor. Sex releases prostaglandins which can stimulate the cervix into action.

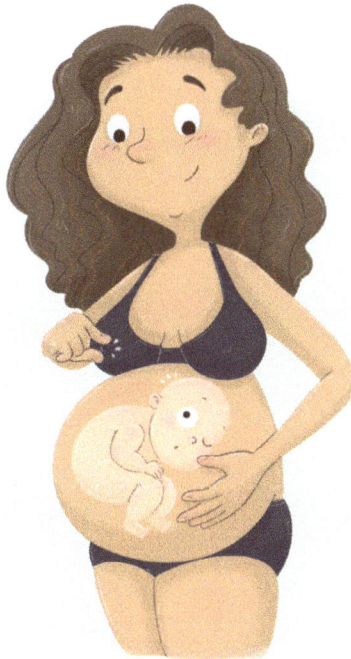

Water Breaking...or Not

Go time: Your water break may be textbook, complete with seeing the mucus plug and 'gush,' or you may have no noticeable signs other than increasingly strong and frequent labor pains.

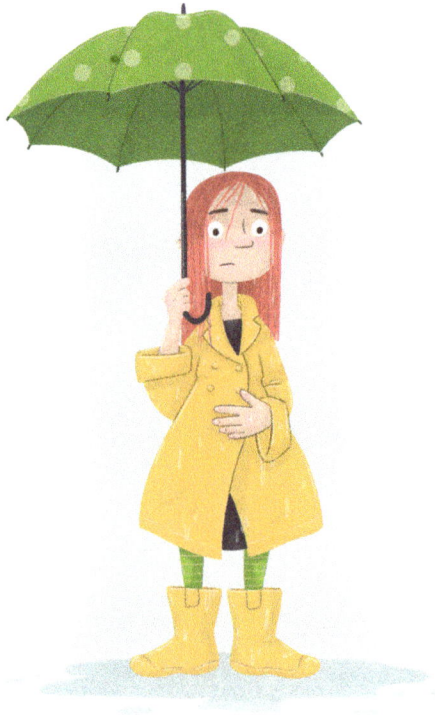

All the Positions

Don't be afraid to move around. There may be more positions for delivering the baby than there were for making the baby. Find what is most comfortable for you.

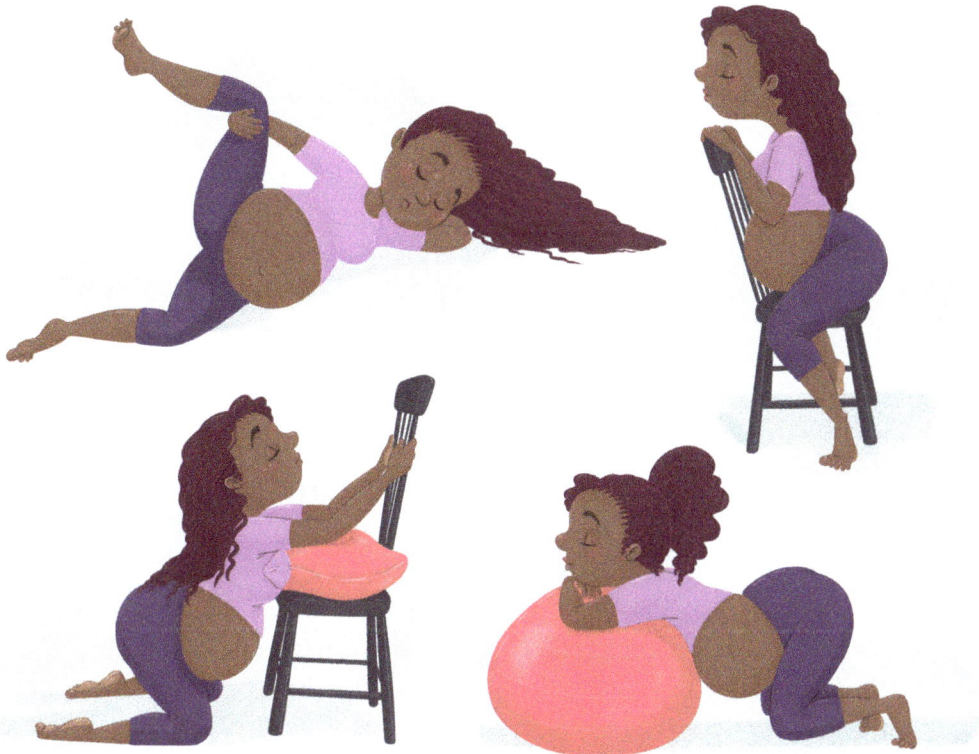

Communicate With Your Team

Talk with your partner, provider, and support team—
Tell them what you want.

Make copies of all important information like, medical information, emergency numbers, allergies, preferences, birth plan.

Keep all this information in an easily accessible spot.

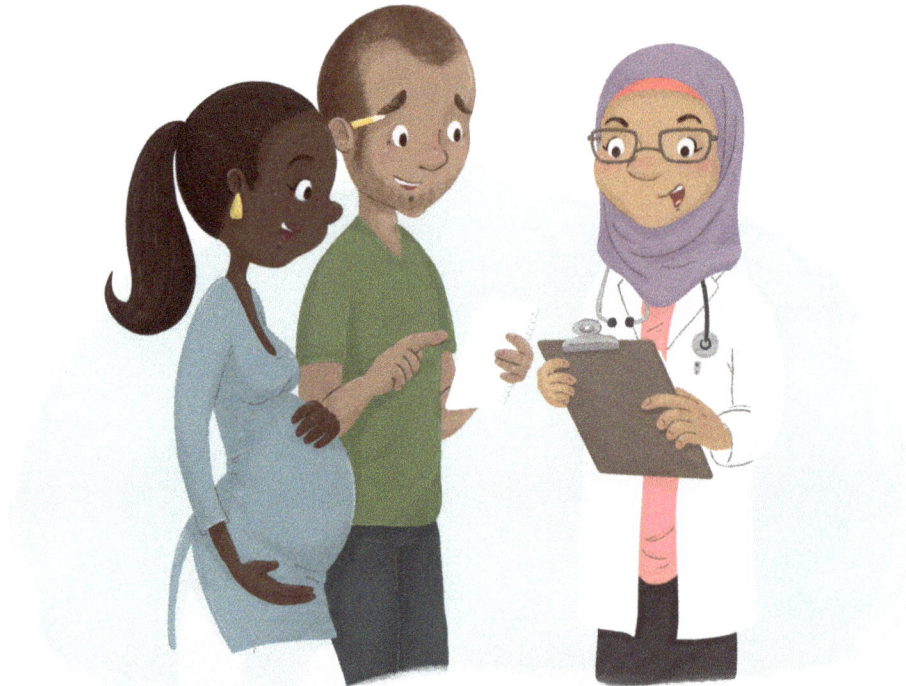

Stigmas and Opinions

Everyone will have an opinion on natural births, epidurals, Pitocin, induction, cesarean births . . . the list goes on.

Ignore the banter and stigmas and do what you and your provider have decided is best for you.

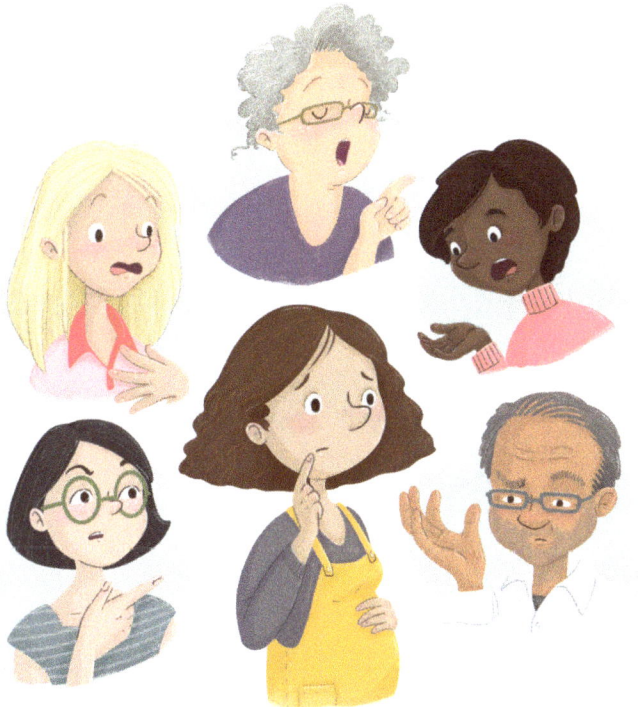

Your Private Property is Now Public Domain

Everyone in the room will see everything,
hear everything, smell everything.

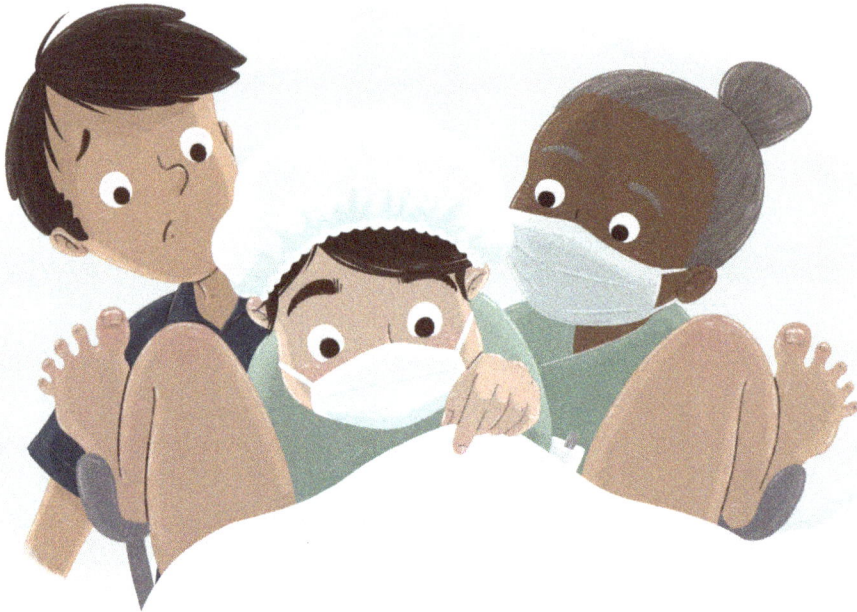

Bodily Fluids...

... will be everywhere.
You may pee, poop, vomit, or all three!

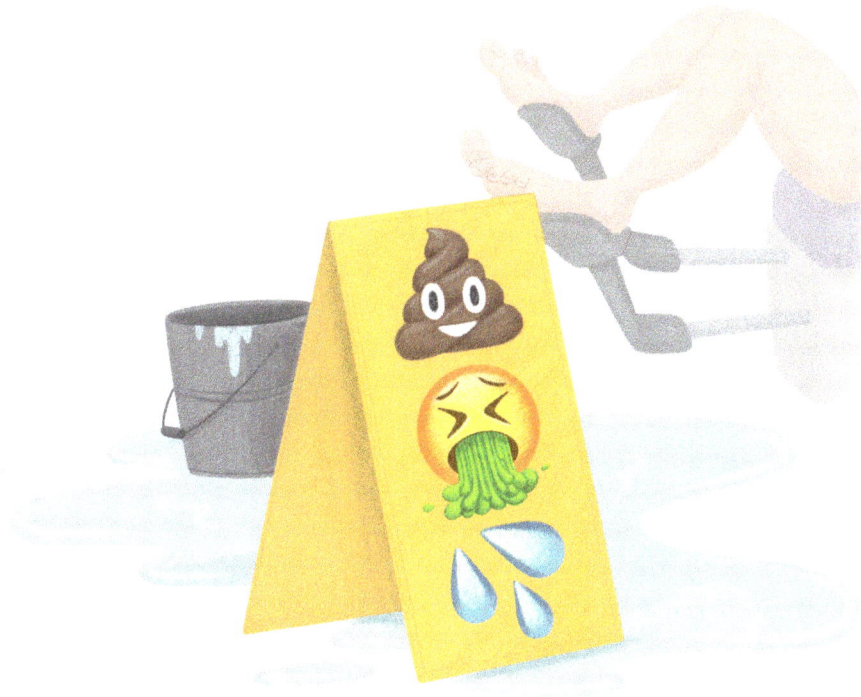

If you have a partner, they may be amazing...

The support, love, and compassion you receive from your significant other may blow you away.

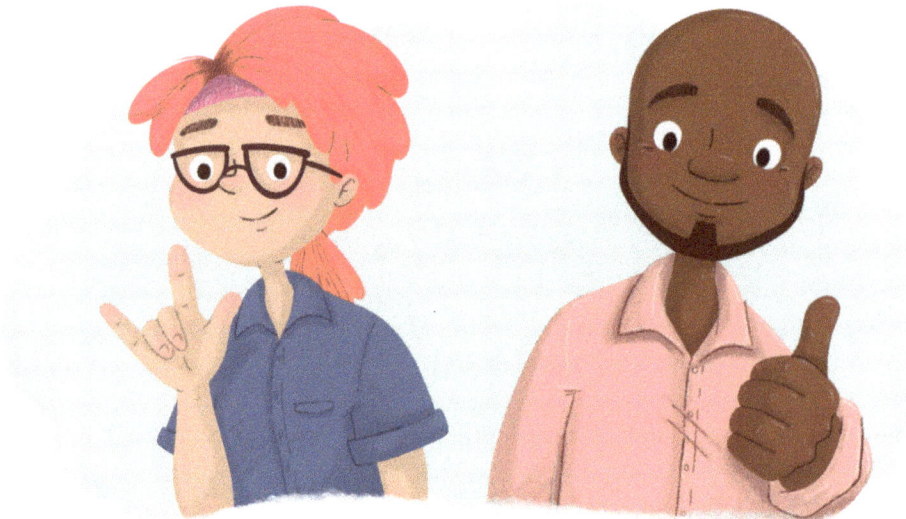

...until they pass out, or have a hard time seeing you in pain

They may get tired, have a hard time seeing you in pain, pass out, or get grossed out!

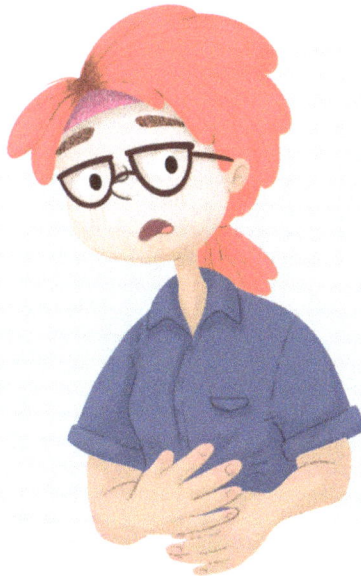

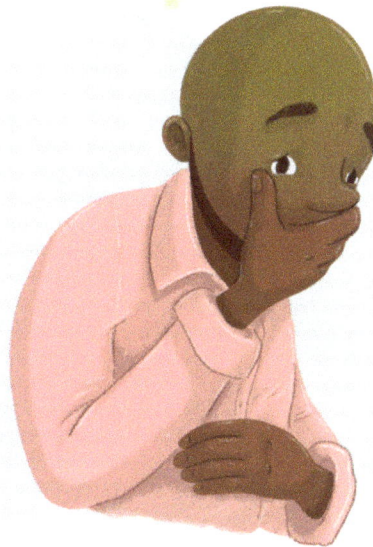

Labor #2 – Placentas

After you deliver your baby, you will deliver your placenta
(aka the afterbirth).

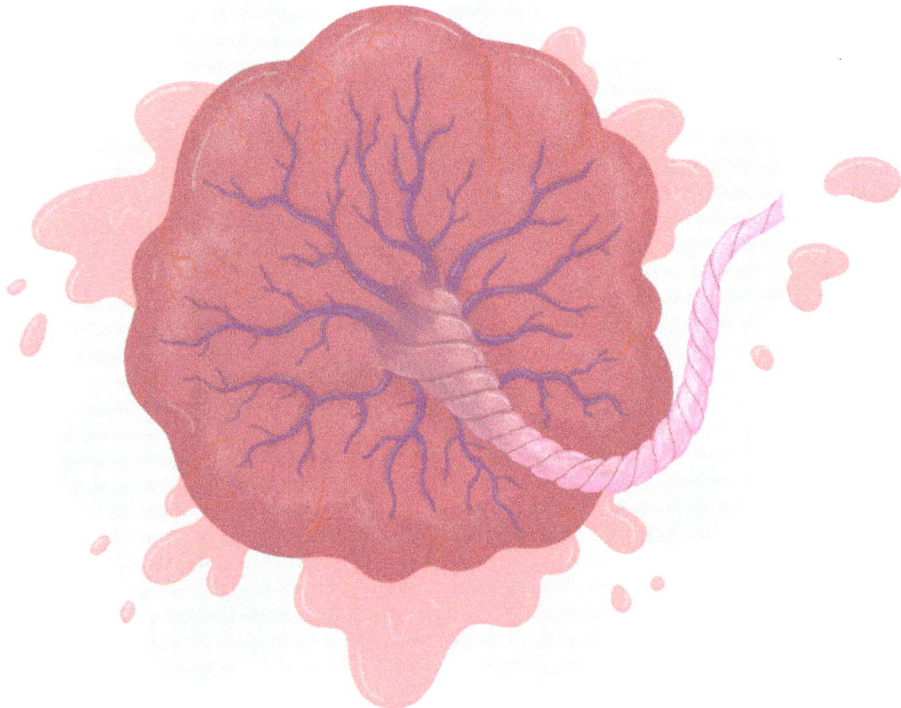

Perineal Tears

There may be tears streaming down your face and tears in the vaginal opening during the delivery. These can range in severity from first to fourth degree. Though rare, if the vaginal opening does not expand rapidly enough the doctor or midwife may perform an episiotomy (or surgical incision) to assist in delivery.

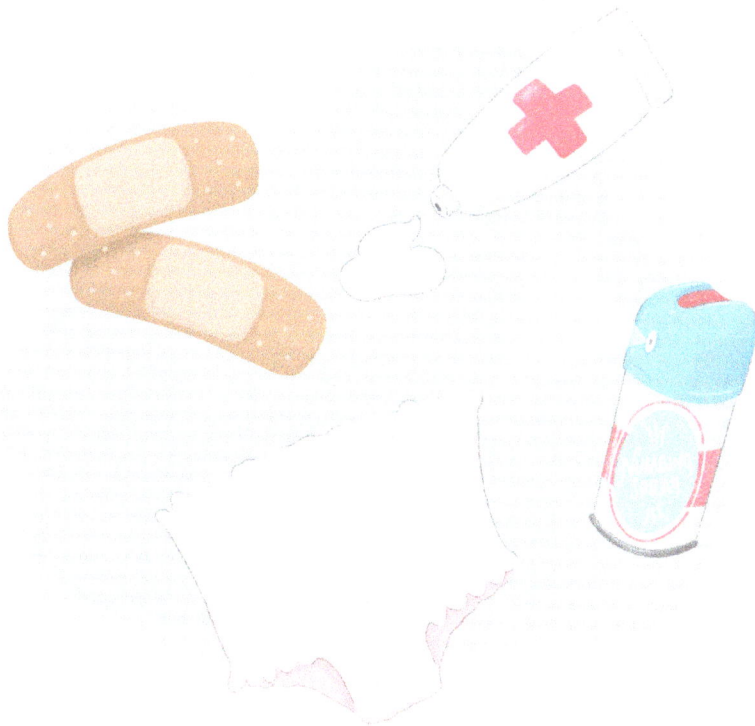

Ice, Ice Baby and Painful Poops

Post-delivery you will be very, very sore.
Packing ice around your sore nether-regions will help to reduce the swelling and pain.

They worked hard—treat them right!

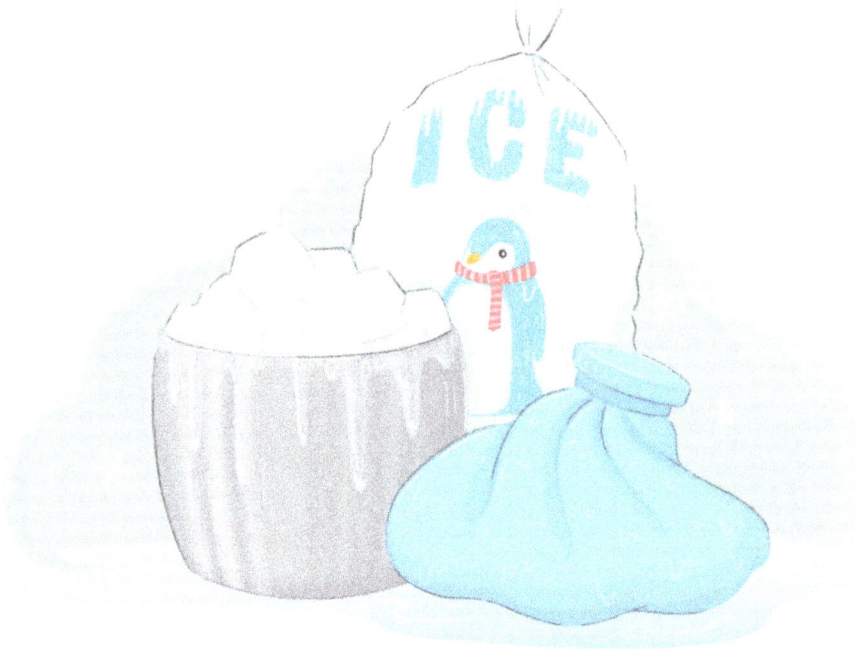

The Ketchup Bottle

After delivery you will receive a special bottle . . . and may wonder where the condiments and hot dog are. It's not for that. It's to help you wash up around your sutures and sores.

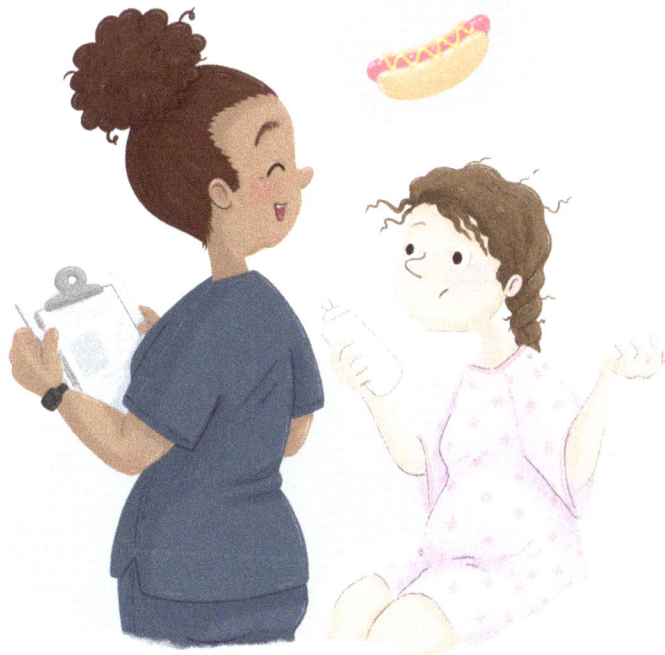

Diapers

Both you and your baby will go home in diapers.
After four to eight weeks, one of you will graduate to
big girl undies!

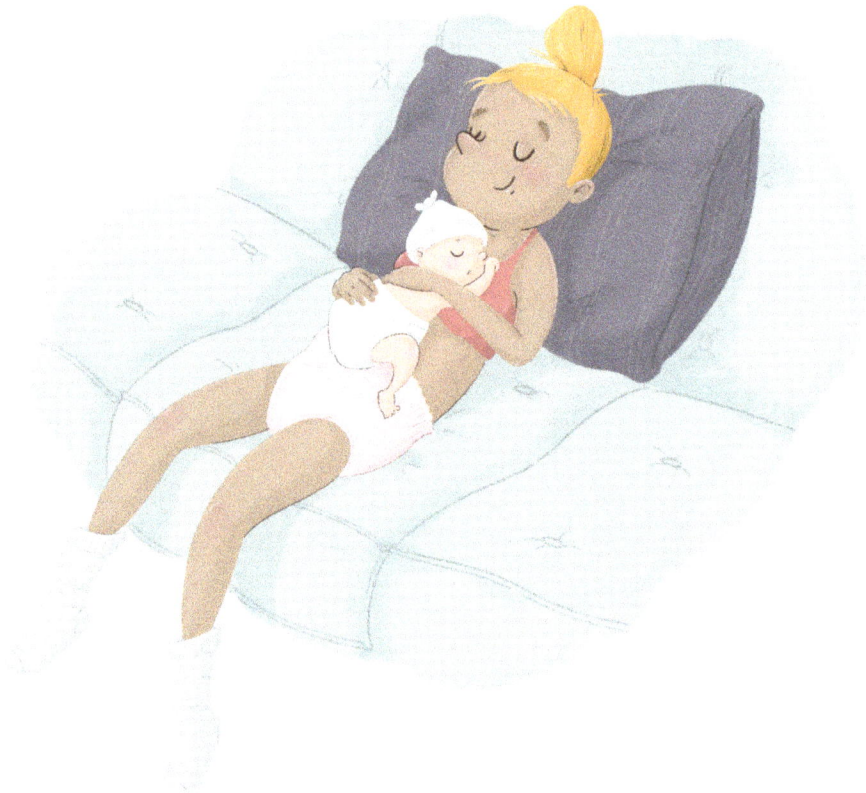

Post-Delivery Time: You Time or Family Time?

Be clear about your time and boundaries after the baby is born. If family and friends would like to come over, have them do a chore to help.

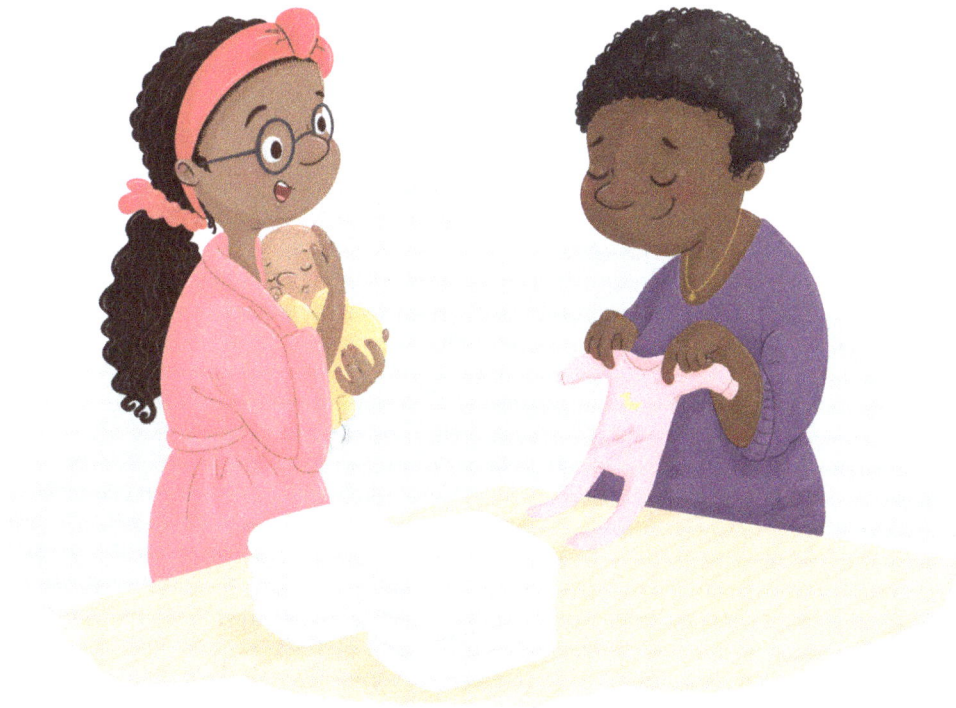

But What About...

When my baby decides to arrive?

- This is unique to each woman and her pregnancy. Your water may break in a gush, or may be just a trickle. You may dilate instantly or slowly. Your baby may arrive with the momentum and passion of Lance Armstrong crossing the finish line, or your baby may creep out with the lethargy of a couch potato on a Saturday afternoon. Some women deliver similarly in each pregnancy, and some do not. It is dependent upon the body and context of each pregnancy and its L&D experience.

Hydration during labor & delivery?

- It is imperative to enter labor well hydrated. Continue drinking as labor and delivery progresses and continue to hydrate in moderate amounts (one cup per hour) until your baby has arrived. Labor and delivery is an intensive exercise and the body needs fuel (food) and hydration (water) to maintain energy, for contractions to remain strong and regular, and the body function properly.

My milk supply?

- It may come as a surprise, but your milk supply will not emerge immediately. For the first two to three days, your baby will drink the colostrum that your body has been producing since around your 20th week of pregnancy. By day three, milk production will increase for most women. Signs to look for are fullness and swelling of the breasts, leaking milk, and changes in feeding. Remember your baby's tummy is tiny at first and will likely not need much, especially in the first few days.

"Breast is Best"?

- Yeah, you've heard it shouted from a mountaintop. Well, we strongly disagree. Our mantra is instead "Fed is Best," for both baby and mom. If breastfeeding is your jam and your body is able to produce and supply enough milk, great! If you choose not to breastfeed or are unable to do so and are using reputable donor milk or a nutritious formula to feed your baby, great! For more moms than I can count and for more reasons than I can recall, breastfeeding simply wasn't an option, and that's okay. At the end of the day the most important thing is that baby is being fed nutritious formula or milk and Momma has the peace of mind to not stress about it. PS: As with everything else, this is not anybody else's business or place to have an opinion. PPS: For support, reach out to your provider, doula, or lactation consultant. If they can't help, they can point to a place or person who can.

Leaving the hospital?

- At the time of the publishing, the standard time to remain in the hospital for a vaginal birth with no complications is one to two days. The standard time to remain in the hospital for a C-section with no complications is two to four days. A lot will happen while you're in the hospital: you and baby will be monitored to evaluate stability and health, any medication and anesthesia given during labor will wear off, tears and bruising will be evaluated, your uterus will be checked and monitored for excess bleeding, you may meet with a lactation consultant, you may take your first shower and learn to clean and care for any tears, and you will be introduced to the postpartum diapers you'll wear for the next few weeks. If you have had a C-section, you will also be monitored to: use the bathroom unassisted, urinate without a catheter, eat and drink unassisted, pass gas, and sit upright. You'll also have your incisions monitored and learn next steps for healing.

Resources:

- Your best resource is a trusted provider. The resources below may help you connect to reliable and reputable doctors, nurse practitioners, midwives, doulas, lactation consultants, and other support and community in your area.

Books:

- *Nine Months or Forty Weeks?: The Shit They Don't Tell You About Pregnancy*, by Carolyn Byrd
- *The Womanly Art of Breastfeeding*, by La Leche League International
- *Good Moms Have Scary Thoughts*, by Karen Kleiman

Online Resources:

- The American College of Obstetricians and Gynecologists www.acog.org/womens-health/pregnancy/labor-and-delivery-

- Share With Women, providing free handouts and articles from The Journal of MidWifery & Women's Health covering a range of topics www.sharewithwomen.org

- Postpartum Support International www.postpartum.net/get-help/

- UNC Perinatal Mood Clinic www.med.unc.edu/psych/wmd/mood-disorders/perinatal/

- 4th Trimester Project www.newmomhealth.com/

- Evidence Based Birth www.evidencebasedbirth.com/

- Evidence Based Birth Podcast www.stitcher.com/show/evidence-based-birthr

About the Author

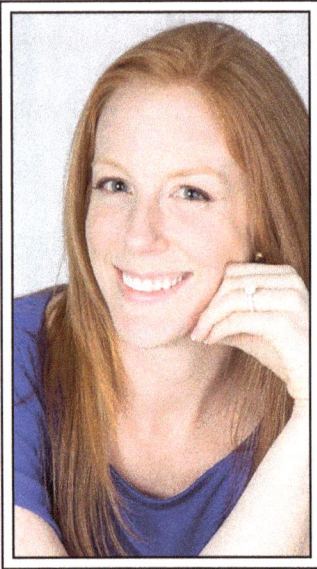

Carolyn Byrd is the owner and founder of Cary Integrative Health, a health care collaborative to mental health providers, dieticians, functional medicine doctors, massage therapists, acupuncturists, and coaches. Within the practice she works as a habit and health coach and massage therapist. She is also a registered yoga teacher, a personal trainer, and veteran. Her work focuses on moving her clients out of mental, habitual, and physical blocks and pain patterns. She is passionate about what she does and believes education and community are keys to optimal health care.

She is wife to Cameron and momma to Cardinal Elizabeth, to whom she holds highest gratitude and love for making her a better person every day. When she is not at her clinic or at home with her people and menagerie of pets, you can find her at the barn riding her horse, Godiva, or cooking up something plant-based and gluten free.

About the Illustrator

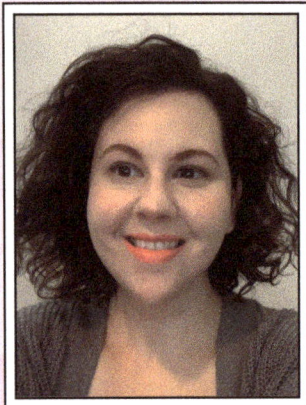

Sarah Gramelspacher worked on the illustrations for this book during her third trimester of pregnancy, while experiencing some—but not all—of the phenomena described in its pages!

Growing up in and around New Orleans, Sarah started drawing as soon as she could hold a crayon, and has never stopped! She studied painting at the University of New Orleans and earned her BA in 2006. Sarah has exhibited paintings in galleries across the U.S., and has created illustrations for picture books, middle-grade novels, and magazines. She has worked with Highlights Magazine, Cricket Media, and Arcadia Publishing, to name a few. She is represented by Kate Kendrick at Astound Agency.

www.ingramcontent.com/pod-product-compliance
Lightning Source LLC
Chambersburg PA
CBHW041604260326
41914CB00012B/1384